In conjunction with **Post Surgery Recovery Diary** this book **Post Surgery Recovery Diary 2** is for individuals wanting additional pages to document medications and statistics. This book contains sixty days of charts for continued daily recovery.

Randy T. Olson

Published through Amazon.com
ISBN-13: **978-1502904416**

Notes

Daily Medication

Date ____/____/____

Medications	Morning	Afternoon	Evening
Drug & Dose:	Time:		
Drug & Dose:			
Drug & Dose:			
Drug & Dose:			
Drug & Dose:			
Drug & Dose:			
Drug & Dose:			

Daily Statistics

Weight:	Temp:	Hours Slept:
Heart rate:	Walking time:	Blood Pressure:
How do you feel (1 being poor) circle: ⟹	**1 2 3 4 5 6 7 8 9 10**	

Notes

Daily Medication

Date ____/____/____

Medications	Morning	Afternoon	Evening
Drug & Dose:	Time:		
Drug & Dose:			
Drug & Dose:			
Drug & Dose:			
Drug & Dose:			
Drug & Dose:			
Drug & Dose:			

Daily Statistics

Weight:	Temp:	Hours Slept:
Heart rate:	Walking time:	Blood Pressure:
How do you feel (1 being poor) circle: ⟹	**1 2 3 4 5 6 7 8 9 10**	

Notes

Daily Medication

Date ____/____/____

Medications	Morning	Afternoon	Evening
Drug & Dose:	Time:		
Drug & Dose:			
Drug & Dose:			
Drug & Dose:			
Drug & Dose:			
Drug & Dose:			
Drug & Dose:			

Daily Statistics

Weight:	Temp:	Hours Slept:
Heart rate:	Walking time:	Blood Pressure:
How do you feel (1 being poor) circle: ⟹	1 2 3 4 5 6 7 8 9 10	

Notes

Daily Medication

Date ____/____/____

Medications	Morning	Afternoon	Evening
Drug & Dose:	Time:		
Drug & Dose:			
Drug & Dose:			
Drug & Dose:			
Drug & Dose:			
Drug & Dose:			
Drug & Dose:			

Daily Statistics

Weight:	Temp:	Hours Slept:
Heart rate:	Walking time:	Blood Pressure:
How do you feel (1 being poor) circle: ⟹	**1 2 3 4 5 6 7 8 9 10**	

Notes

Daily Medication

Date ____/____/____

Medications		Morning	Afternoon	Evening
Drug & Dose:		Time:		
Drug & Dose:				
Drug & Dose:				
Drug & Dose:				
Drug & Dose:				
Drug & Dose:				
Drug & Dose:				

Daily Statistics

Weight:	Temp:	Hours Slept:
Heart rate:	Walking time:	Blood Pressure:
How do you feel (1 being poor) circle: ⟹	**1 2 3 4 5 6 7 8 9 10**	

Notes

Daily Medication

Date ____/____/____

Medications	Morning	Afternoon	Evening
Drug & Dose:	Time:		
Drug & Dose:			
Drug & Dose:			
Drug & Dose:			
Drug & Dose:			
Drug & Dose:			
Drug & Dose:			

Daily Statistics

Weight:	Temp:	Hours Slept:
Heart rate:	Walking time:	Blood Pressure:
How do you feel (1 being poor) circle: ⟹	**1 2 3 4 5 6 7 8 9 10**	

Notes

Daily Medication

Date ____/____/____

Medications	Morning	Afternoon	Evening
Drug & Dose:	Time:		
Drug & Dose:			
Drug & Dose:			
Drug & Dose:			
Drug & Dose:			
Drug & Dose:			
Drug & Dose:			

Daily Statistics

Weight:	Temp:	Hours Slept:
Heart rate:	Walking time:	Blood Pressure:
How do you feel (1 being poor) circle: ⟹	1 2 3 4 5 6 7 8 9 10	

Notes

Daily Medication

Date ____/____/____

Medications	Morning	Afternoon	Evening
Drug & Dose:	Time:		
Drug & Dose:			
Drug & Dose:			
Drug & Dose:			
Drug & Dose:			
Drug & Dose:			
Drug & Dose:			

Daily Statistics

Weight:	Temp:	Hours Slept:
Heart rate:	Walking time:	Blood Pressure:
How do you feel (1 being poor) circle: ⟹	**1 2 3 4 5 6 7 8 9 10**	

Notes

Daily Medication

Date ____/____/____

Medications	Morning	Afternoon	Evening
Drug & Dose:	Time:		
Drug & Dose:			
Drug & Dose:			
Drug & Dose:			
Drug & Dose:			
Drug & Dose:			
Drug & Dose:			

Daily Statistics

Weight:	Temp:	Hours Slept:
Heart rate:	Walking time:	Blood Pressure:
How do you feel (1 being poor) circle: ⟹	**1 2 3 4 5 6 7 8 9 10**	

Notes

Daily Medication

Date ____/____/____

Medications	Morning	Afternoon	Evening
Drug & Dose:	Time:		
Drug & Dose:			
Drug & Dose:			
Drug & Dose:			
Drug & Dose:			
Drug & Dose:			
Drug & Dose:			

Daily Statistics

Weight:	Temp:	Hours Slept:
Heart rate:	Walking time:	Blood Pressure:
How do you feel (1 being poor) circle: ⟹	**1 2 3 4 5 6 7 8 9 10**	

Notes

Daily Medication

Date ____/____/____

Medications	Morning	Afternoon	Evening
Drug & Dose:	Time:		
Drug & Dose:			
Drug & Dose:			
Drug & Dose:			
Drug & Dose:			
Drug & Dose:			
Drug & Dose:			

Daily Statistics

Weight:	Temp:	Hours Slept:
Heart rate:	Walking time:	Blood Pressure:
How do you feel (1 being poor) circle: ⟹	**1 2 3 4 5 6 7 8 9 10**	

Notes

Daily Medication

Date ____/____/____

Medications	Morning	Afternoon	Evening
Drug & Dose:	Time:		
Drug & Dose:			
Drug & Dose:			
Drug & Dose:			
Drug & Dose:			
Drug & Dose:			
Drug & Dose:			

Daily Statistics

Weight:	Temp:	Hours Slept:
Heart rate:	Walking time:	Blood Pressure:
How do you feel (1 being poor) circle: ⟹	**1 2 3 4 5 6 7 8 9 10**	

27

Notes

Daily Medication

Date ____/____/____

Medications	Morning	Afternoon	Evening
Drug & Dose:	Time:		
Drug & Dose:			
Drug & Dose:			
Drug & Dose:			
Drug & Dose:			
Drug & Dose:			
Drug & Dose:			

Daily Statistics

Weight:	Temp:	Hours Slept:
Heart rate:	Walking time:	Blood Pressure:
How do you feel (1 being poor) circle:	1 2 3 4 5 6 7 8 9 10	

Notes

Daily Medication

Date ____/____/____

Medications	Morning	Afternoon	Evening
Drug & Dose:	Time:		
Drug & Dose:			
Drug & Dose:			
Drug & Dose:			
Drug & Dose:			
Drug & Dose:			
Drug & Dose:			

Daily Statistics

Weight:	Temp:	Hours Slept:
Heart rate:	Walking time:	Blood Pressure:
How do you feel (1 being poor) circle:	**1 2 3 4 5 6 7 8 9 10**	

Notes

Daily Medication

Date ____/____/____

Medications	Morning	Afternoon	Evening
Drug & Dose:	Time:		
Drug & Dose:			
Drug & Dose:			
Drug & Dose:			
Drug & Dose:			
Drug & Dose:			
Drug & Dose:			

Daily Statistics

Weight:	Temp:	Hours Slept:
Heart rate:	Walking time:	Blood Pressure:
How do you feel (1 being poor) circle: ⟹	**1 2 3 4 5 6 7 8 9 10**	

Notes

Daily Medication

Date ____ / ____ / ____

Medications		Morning	Afternoon	Evening
Drug & Dose:		Time:		
Drug & Dose:				
Drug & Dose:				
Drug & Dose:				
Drug & Dose:				
Drug & Dose:				
Drug & Dose:				

Daily Statistics

Weight:	Temp:	Hours Slept:
Heart rate:	Walking time:	Blood Pressure:
How do you feel (1 being poor) circle: ⟹	**1 2 3 4 5 6 7 8 9 10**	

Notes

Daily Medication

Date ____/____/____

Medications	Morning	Afternoon	Evening
Drug & Dose:	Time:		
Drug & Dose:			
Drug & Dose:			
Drug & Dose:			
Drug & Dose:			
Drug & Dose:			
Drug & Dose:			

Daily Statistics

Weight:	Temp:	Hours Slept:
Heart rate:	Walking time:	Blood Pressure:
How do you feel (1 being poor) circle: ⟹	**1 2 3 4 5 6 7 8 9 10**	

Notes

Daily Medication

Date ____/____/____

Medications	Morning	Afternoon	Evening
Drug & Dose:	Time:		
Drug & Dose:			
Drug & Dose:			
Drug & Dose:			
Drug & Dose:			
Drug & Dose:			
Drug & Dose:			

Daily Statistics

Weight:	Temp:	Hours Slept:
Heart rate:	Walking time:	Blood Pressure:
How do you feel (1 being poor) circle: ⟹	**1 2 3 4 5 6 7 8 9 10**	

Notes

Daily Medication

Date ____/____/____

Medications	Morning	Afternoon	Evening
Drug & Dose:	Time:		
Drug & Dose:			
Drug & Dose:			
Drug & Dose:			
Drug & Dose:			
Drug & Dose:			
Drug & Dose:			

Daily Statistics

Weight:	Temp:	Hours Slept:
Heart rate:	Walking time:	Blood Pressure:
How do you feel (1 being poor) circle: ⟹	**1 2 3 4 5 6 7 8 9 10**	

Notes

Daily Medication

Date ____/____/____

Medications	Morning	Afternoon	Evening
Drug & Dose:	Time:		
Drug & Dose:			
Drug & Dose:			
Drug & Dose:			
Drug & Dose:			
Drug & Dose:			
Drug & Dose:			

Daily Statistics

Weight:	Temp:	Hours Slept:
Heart rate:	Walking time:	Blood Pressure:
How do you feel (1 being poor) circle:	**1 2 3 4 5 6 7 8 9 10**	

Notes

Daily Medication

Date ____/____/____

Medications		Morning	Afternoon	Evening
Drug & Dose:		Time:		
Drug & Dose:				
Drug & Dose:				
Drug & Dose:				
Drug & Dose:				
Drug & Dose:				
Drug & Dose:				

Daily Statistics

Weight:	Temp:	Hours Slept:
Heart rate:	Walking time:	Blood Pressure:
How do you feel (1 being poor) circle: ⟹	**1 2 3 4 5 6 7 8 9 10**	

Notes

Daily Medication

Date ____/____/____

Medications		Morning	Afternoon	Evening
Drug & Dose:		Time:		
Drug & Dose:				
Drug & Dose:				
Drug & Dose:				
Drug & Dose:				
Drug & Dose:				
Drug & Dose:				

Daily Statistics

Weight:	Temp:	Hours Slept:
Heart rate:	Walking time:	Blood Pressure:
How do you feel (1 being poor) circle: ⟹	**1 2 3 4 5 6 7 8 9 10**	

Notes

Daily Medication

Date ____/____/____

Medications	Morning	Afternoon	Evening
Drug & Dose:	Time:		
Drug & Dose:			
Drug & Dose:			
Drug & Dose:			
Drug & Dose:			
Drug & Dose:			
Drug & Dose:			

Daily Statistics

Weight:	Temp:	Hours Slept:
Heart rate:	Walking time:	Blood Pressure:
How do you feel (1 being poor) circle: ⟹	**1 2 3 4 5 6 7 8 9 10**	

Notes

Daily Medication

Date _____ / _____ / _____

Medications	Morning	Afternoon	Evening
Drug & Dose:	Time:		
Drug & Dose:			
Drug & Dose:			
Drug & Dose:			
Drug & Dose:			
Drug & Dose:			
Drug & Dose:			

Daily Statistics

Weight:	Temp:	Hours Slept:
Heart rate:	Walking time:	Blood Pressure:
How do you feel (1 being poor) circle: ⟹	**1 2 3 4 5 6 7 8 9 10**	

Notes

Daily Medication

Date ____/____/____

Medications	Morning	Afternoon	Evening
Drug & Dose:	Time:		
Drug & Dose:			
Drug & Dose:			
Drug & Dose:			
Drug & Dose:			
Drug & Dose:			
Drug & Dose:			

Daily Statistics

Weight:	Temp:	Hours Slept:
Heart rate:	Walking time:	Blood Pressure:
How do you feel (1 being poor) circle: ⟹	**1 2 3 4 5 6 7 8 9 10**	

Notes

Daily Medication

Date ____/____/____

Medications		Morning	Afternoon	Evening
Drug & Dose:		Time:		
Drug & Dose:				
Drug & Dose:				
Drug & Dose:				
Drug & Dose:				
Drug & Dose:				
Drug & Dose:				

Daily Statistics

Weight:	Temp:	Hours Slept:
Heart rate:	Walking time:	Blood Pressure:
How do you feel (1 being poor) circle: ⟹	**1 2 3 4 5 6 7 8 9 10**	

Notes

Daily Medication

Date ____/____/____

Medications	Morning	Afternoon	Evening
Drug & Dose:	Time:		
Drug & Dose:			
Drug & Dose:			
Drug & Dose:			
Drug & Dose:			
Drug & Dose:			
Drug & Dose:			

Daily Statistics

Weight:	Temp:	Hours Slept:
Heart rate:	Walking time:	Blood Pressure:
How do you feel (1 being poor) circle:	1 2 3 4 5 6 7 8 9 10	

Notes

Daily Medication

Date ____/____/____

Medications	Morning	Afternoon	Evening
Drug & Dose:	Time:		
Drug & Dose:			
Drug & Dose:			
Drug & Dose:			
Drug & Dose:			
Drug & Dose:			
Drug & Dose:			

Daily Statistics

Weight:	Temp:	Hours Slept:
Heart rate:	Walking time:	Blood Pressure:
How do you feel (1 being poor) circle: ⟹	**1 2 3 4 5 6 7 8 9 10**	

Notes

Daily Medication

Date ____/____/____

Medications	Morning	Afternoon	Evening
Drug & Dose:	Time:		
Drug & Dose:			
Drug & Dose:			
Drug & Dose:			
Drug & Dose:			
Drug & Dose:			
Drug & Dose:			

Daily Statistics

Weight:	Temp:	Hours Slept:
Heart rate:	Walking time:	Blood Pressure:
How do you feel (1 being poor) circle: ⟹	**1 2 3 4 5 6 7 8 9 10**	

Notes

Daily Medication

Date ____/____/____

Medications	Morning	Afternoon	Evening
Drug & Dose:	Time:		
Drug & Dose:			
Drug & Dose:			
Drug & Dose:			
Drug & Dose:			
Drug & Dose:			
Drug & Dose:			

Daily Statistics

Weight:	Temp:	Hours Slept:
Heart rate:	Walking time:	Blood Pressure:
How do you feel (1 being poor) circle: ⟹	**1 2 3 4 5 6 7 8 9 10**	

Notes

Daily Medication

Date ____/____/____

Medications	Morning	Afternoon	Evening
Drug & Dose:	Time:		
Drug & Dose:			
Drug & Dose:			
Drug & Dose:			
Drug & Dose:			
Drug & Dose:			
Drug & Dose:			

Daily Statistics

Weight:	Temp:	Hours Slept:
Heart rate:	Walking time:	Blood Pressure:
How do you feel (1 being poor) circle: ⟹	**1 2 3 4 5 6 7 8 9 10**	

Notes

Daily Medication

Date ____/____/____

Medications	Morning	Afternoon	Evening
Drug & Dose:	Time:		
Drug & Dose:			
Drug & Dose:			
Drug & Dose:			
Drug & Dose:			
Drug & Dose:			
Drug & Dose:			

Daily Statistics

Weight:	Temp:	Hours Slept:
Heart rate:	Walking time:	Blood Pressure:
How do you feel (1 being poor) circle: ⟹	**1 2 3 4 5 6 7 8 9 10**	

Notes

Daily Medication

Date ____/____/____

Medications	Morning	Afternoon	Evening
Drug & Dose:	Time:		
Drug & Dose:			
Drug & Dose:			
Drug & Dose:			
Drug & Dose:			
Drug & Dose:			
Drug & Dose:			

Daily Statistics

Weight:	Temp:	Hours Slept:
Heart rate:	Walking time:	Blood Pressure:
How do you feel (1 being poor) circle: ⟹	**1 2 3 4 5 6 7 8 9 10**	

Notes

Daily Medication

Date _____/_____/_____

Medications	Morning	Afternoon	Evening
Drug & Dose:	Time:		
Drug & Dose:			
Drug & Dose:			
Drug & Dose:			
Drug & Dose:			
Drug & Dose:			
Drug & Dose:			

Daily Statistics

Weight:	Temp:	Hours Slept:
Heart rate:	Walking time:	Blood Pressure:
How do you feel (1 being poor) circle: ⟹	**1 2 3 4 5 6 7 8 9 10**	

Notes

Daily Medication

Date ____/____/____

Medications		Morning	Afternoon	Evening
Drug & Dose:		Time:		
Drug & Dose:				
Drug & Dose:				
Drug & Dose:				
Drug & Dose:				
Drug & Dose:				
Drug & Dose:				

Daily Statistics

Weight:	Temp:	Hours Slept:
Heart rate:	Walking time:	Blood Pressure:
How do you feel (1 being poor) circle: ⟹	**1 2 3 4 5 6 7 8 9 10**	

Notes

Daily Medication

Date ____/____/____

Medications	Morning	Afternoon	Evening
Drug & Dose:	Time:		
Drug & Dose:			
Drug & Dose:			
Drug & Dose:			
Drug & Dose:			
Drug & Dose:			
Drug & Dose:			

Daily Statistics

Weight:	Temp:	Hours Slept:
Heart rate:	Walking time:	Blood Pressure:
How do you feel (1 being poor) circle:	**1 2 3 4 5 6 7 8 9 10**	

Notes

Daily Medication

Date ____/____/____

Medications	Morning	Afternoon	Evening
Drug & Dose:	Time:		
Drug & Dose:			
Drug & Dose:			
Drug & Dose:			
Drug & Dose:			
Drug & Dose:			
Drug & Dose:			

Daily Statistics

Weight:	Temp:	Hours Slept:
Heart rate:	Walking time:	Blood Pressure:
How do you feel (1 being poor) circle: ⟹	**1 2 3 4 5 6 7 8 9 10**	

Notes

Daily Medication

Date ____/____/____

Medications	Morning	Afternoon	Evening
Drug & Dose:	Time:		
Drug & Dose:			
Drug & Dose:			
Drug & Dose:			
Drug & Dose:			
Drug & Dose:			
Drug & Dose:			

Daily Statistics

Weight:	Temp:	Hours Slept:
Heart rate:	Walking time:	Blood Pressure:
How do you feel (1 being poor) circle: ⟹	**1 2 3 4 5 6 7 8 9 10**	

Notes

Daily Medication

Date ____/____/____

Medications	Morning	Afternoon	Evening
Drug & Dose:	Time:		
Drug & Dose:			
Drug & Dose:			
Drug & Dose:			
Drug & Dose:			
Drug & Dose:			
Drug & Dose:			

Daily Statistics

Weight:	Temp:	Hours Slept:
Heart rate:	Walking time:	Blood Pressure:
How do you feel (1 being poor) circle: ⟹	**1 2 3 4 5 6 7 8 9 10**	

Notes

Daily Medication

Date ____/____/____

Medications	Morning	Afternoon	Evening
Drug & Dose:	Time:		
Drug & Dose:			
Drug & Dose:			
Drug & Dose:			
Drug & Dose:			
Drug & Dose:			
Drug & Dose:			

Daily Statistics

Weight:	Temp:	Hours Slept:
Heart rate:	Walking time:	Blood Pressure:
How do you feel (1 being poor) circle:	**1 2 3 4 5 6 7 8 9 10**	

Notes

Daily Medication

Date ____/____/____

Medications	Morning	Afternoon	Evening
Drug & Dose:	Time:		
Drug & Dose:			
Drug & Dose:			
Drug & Dose:			
Drug & Dose:			
Drug & Dose:			
Drug & Dose:			

Daily Statistics

Weight:	Temp:	Hours Slept:
Heart rate:	Walking time:	Blood Pressure:
How do you feel (1 being poor) circle: ⟹	**1 2 3 4 5 6 7 8 9 10**	

Notes

Daily Medication

Date ____/____/____

Medications	Morning	Afternoon	Evening
Drug & Dose:	Time:		
Drug & Dose:			
Drug & Dose:			
Drug & Dose:			
Drug & Dose:			
Drug & Dose:			
Drug & Dose:			

Daily Statistics

Weight:	Temp:	Hours Slept:
Heart rate:	Walking time:	Blood Pressure:
How do you feel (1 being poor) circle: ⟹	**1 2 3 4 5 6 7 8 9 10**	

Notes

Daily Medication

Date ____/____/____

Medications	Morning	Afternoon	Evening
Drug & Dose:	Time:		
Drug & Dose:			
Drug & Dose:			
Drug & Dose:			
Drug & Dose:			
Drug & Dose:			
Drug & Dose:			

Daily Statistics

Weight:	Temp:	Hours Slept:
Heart rate:	Walking time:	Blood Pressure:
How do you feel (1 being poor) circle: ⟹	**1 2 3 4 5 6 7 8 9 10**	

Notes

Daily Medication

Date ____/____/____

Medications		Morning	Afternoon	Evening
Drug & Dose:		Time:		
Drug & Dose:				
Drug & Dose:				
Drug & Dose:				
Drug & Dose:				
Drug & Dose:				
Drug & Dose:				

Daily Statistics

Weight:	Temp:	Hours Slept:
Heart rate:	Walking time:	Blood Pressure:
How do you feel (1 being poor) circle: ⟹	**1 2 3 4 5 6 7 8 9 10**	

Notes

Daily Medication

Date ____ / ____ / ____

Medications	Morning	Afternoon	Evening
Drug & Dose:	Time:		
Drug & Dose:			
Drug & Dose:			
Drug & Dose:			
Drug & Dose:			
Drug & Dose:			
Drug & Dose:			

Daily Statistics

Weight:	Temp:	Hours Slept:
Heart rate:	Walking time:	Blood Pressure:
How do you feel (1 being poor) circle: ⟹	**1 2 3 4 5 6 7 8 9 10**	

Notes

Daily Medication

Date ____/____/____

Medications	Morning	Afternoon	Evening
Drug & Dose:	Time:		
Drug & Dose:			
Drug & Dose:			
Drug & Dose:			
Drug & Dose:			
Drug & Dose:			
Drug & Dose:			

Daily Statistics

Weight:	Temp:	Hours Slept:
Heart rate:	Walking time:	Blood Pressure:
How do you feel (1 being poor) circle: ⟹	**1 2 3 4 5 6 7 8 9 10**	

Notes

Daily Medication

Date ____/____/____

Medications		Morning	Afternoon	Evening
Drug & Dose:		Time:		
Drug & Dose:				
Drug & Dose:				
Drug & Dose:				
Drug & Dose:				
Drug & Dose:				
Drug & Dose:				

Daily Statistics

Weight:	Temp:	Hours Slept:
Heart rate:	Walking time:	Blood Pressure:
How do you feel (1 being poor) circle: ⟹	**1 2 3 4 5 6 7 8 9 10**	

Notes

Daily Medication

Date ____ / ____ / ____

Medications		Morning	Afternoon	Evening
Drug & Dose:		Time:		
Drug & Dose:				
Drug & Dose:				
Drug & Dose:				
Drug & Dose:				
Drug & Dose:				
Drug & Dose:				

Daily Statistics

Weight:	Temp:	Hours Slept:
Heart rate:	Walking time:	Blood Pressure:
How do you feel (1 being poor) circle: ⟹	**1 2 3 4 5 6 7 8 9 10**	

Notes

Daily Medication

Date ____/____/____

Medications	Morning	Afternoon	Evening
Drug & Dose:	Time:		
Drug & Dose:			
Drug & Dose:			
Drug & Dose:			
Drug & Dose:			
Drug & Dose:			
Drug & Dose:			

Daily Statistics

Weight:	Temp:	Hours Slept:
Heart rate:	Walking time:	Blood Pressure:
How do you feel (1 being poor) circle:	**1 2 3 4 5 6 7 8 9 10**	

Notes

Daily Medication

Date ____/____/____

Medications	Morning	Afternoon	Evening
Drug & Dose:	Time:		
Drug & Dose:			
Drug & Dose:			
Drug & Dose:			
Drug & Dose:			
Drug & Dose:			
Drug & Dose:			

Daily Statistics

Weight:	Temp:	Hours Slept:
Heart rate:	Walking time:	Blood Pressure:
How do you feel (1 being poor) circle: ⟹	**1 2 3 4 5 6 7 8 9 10**	

Notes

Daily Medication

Date ____/____/____

Medications	Morning	Afternoon	Evening
Drug & Dose:	Time:		
Drug & Dose:			
Drug & Dose:			
Drug & Dose:			
Drug & Dose:			
Drug & Dose:			
Drug & Dose:			

Daily Statistics

Weight:	Temp:	Hours Slept:
Heart rate:	Walking time:	Blood Pressure:
How do you feel (1 being poor) circle: ⟹	**1 2 3 4 5 6 7 8 9 10**	

Notes

Daily Medication

Date ____/____/____

Medications		Morning	Afternoon	Evening
Drug & Dose:		Time:		
Drug & Dose:				
Drug & Dose:				
Drug & Dose:				
Drug & Dose:				
Drug & Dose:				
Drug & Dose:				

Daily Statistics

Weight:	Temp:	Hours Slept:
Heart rate:	Walking time:	Blood Pressure:
How do you feel (1 being poor) circle: ⟹	**1 2 3 4 5 6 7 8 9 10**	

Notes

Daily Medication

Date ____ / ____ / ____

Medications	Morning	Afternoon	Evening
Drug & Dose:	Time:		
Drug & Dose:			
Drug & Dose:			
Drug & Dose:			
Drug & Dose:			
Drug & Dose:			
Drug & Dose:			

Daily Statistics

Weight:	Temp:	Hours Slept:
Heart rate:	Walking time:	Blood Pressure:
How do you feel (1 being poor) circle: ⟹	**1 2 3 4 5 6 7 8 9 10**	

Notes

Daily Medication

Date ____/____/____

Medications	Morning	Afternoon	Evening
Drug & Dose:	Time:		
Drug & Dose:			
Drug & Dose:			
Drug & Dose:			
Drug & Dose:			
Drug & Dose:			
Drug & Dose:			

Daily Statistics

Weight:	Temp:	Hours Slept:
Heart rate:	Walking time:	Blood Pressure:
How do you feel (1 being poor) circle: ⟹	**1 2 3 4 5 6 7 8 9 10**	

Notes

Daily Medication

Date ____/____/____

Medications	Morning	Afternoon	Evening
Drug & Dose:	Time:		
Drug & Dose:			
Drug & Dose:			
Drug & Dose:			
Drug & Dose:			
Drug & Dose:			
Drug & Dose:			

Daily Statistics

Weight:	Temp:	Hours Slept:
Heart rate:	Walking time:	Blood Pressure:
How do you feel (1 being poor) circle: ⟹	**1 2 3 4 5 6 7 8 9 10**	

Notes

Daily Medication

Date ____/____/____

Medications	Morning	Afternoon	Evening
Drug & Dose:	Time:		
Drug & Dose:			
Drug & Dose:			
Drug & Dose:			
Drug & Dose:			
Drug & Dose:			
Drug & Dose:			

Daily Statistics

Weight:	Temp:	Hours Slept:
Heart rate:	Walking time:	Blood Pressure:
How do you feel (1 being poor) circle: ⟹	**1 2 3 4 5 6 7 8 9 10**	

Notes

Daily Medication

Date ____/____/____

Medications	Morning	Afternoon	Evening
Drug & Dose:	Time:		
Drug & Dose:			
Drug & Dose:			
Drug & Dose:			
Drug & Dose:			
Drug & Dose:			
Drug & Dose:			

Daily Statistics

Weight:	Temp:	Hours Slept:
Heart rate:	Walking time:	Blood Pressure:
How do you feel ⟹ (1 being poor) circle:	**1 2 3 4 5 6 7 8 9 10**	

Notes

Daily Medication

Date ____/____/____

Medications		Morning	Afternoon	Evening
Drug & Dose:		Time:		
Drug & Dose:				
Drug & Dose:				
Drug & Dose:				
Drug & Dose:				
Drug & Dose:				
Drug & Dose:				

Daily Statistics

Weight:	Temp:	Hours Slept:
Heart rate:	Walking time:	Blood Pressure:
How do you feel (1 being poor) circle: ⟹	**1 2 3 4 5 6 7 8 9 10**	

Notes

Daily Medication

Date ____/____/____

Medications	Morning	Afternoon	Evening
Drug & Dose:	Time:		
Drug & Dose:			
Drug & Dose:			
Drug & Dose:			
Drug & Dose:			
Drug & Dose:			
Drug & Dose:			

Daily Statistics

Weight:	Temp:	Hours Slept:
Heart rate:	Walking time:	Blood Pressure:
How do you feel (1 being poor) circle: ⟹	**1 2 3 4 5 6 7 8 9 10**	

Notes

Daily Medication

Date ____/____/____

Medications	Morning	Afternoon	Evening
Drug & Dose:	Time:		
Drug & Dose:			
Drug & Dose:			
Drug & Dose:			
Drug & Dose:			
Drug & Dose:			
Drug & Dose:			

Daily Statistics

Weight:	Temp:	Hours Slept:
Heart rate:	Walking time:	Blood Pressure:
How do you feel (1 being poor) circle: ⟹	**1 2 3 4 5 6 7 8 9 10**	

Notes

Daily Medication

Date ____/____/____

Medications		Morning	Afternoon	Evening
Drug & Dose:		Time:		
Drug & Dose:				
Drug & Dose:				
Drug & Dose:				
Drug & Dose:				
Drug & Dose:				
Drug & Dose:				

Daily Statistics

Weight:	Temp:	Hours Slept:
Heart rate:	Walking time:	Blood Pressure:
How do you feel (1 being poor) circle: ⟹	**1 2 3 4 5 6 7 8 9 10**	

Notes

Daily Medication

Date ____/____/____

Medications		Morning	Afternoon	Evening
Drug & Dose:		Time:		
Drug & Dose:				
Drug & Dose:				
Drug & Dose:				
Drug & Dose:				
Drug & Dose:				
Drug & Dose:				

Daily Statistics

Weight:	Temp:	Hours Slept:
Heart rate:	Walking time:	Blood Pressure:
How do you feel (1 being poor) circle: ⟹	**1 2 3 4 5 6 7 8 9 10**	

Notes

Daily Medication

Date ____/____/____

Medications		Morning	Afternoon	Evening
Drug & Dose:		Time:		
Drug & Dose:				
Drug & Dose:				
Drug & Dose:				
Drug & Dose:				
Drug & Dose:				
Drug & Dose:				

Daily Statistics

Weight:	Temp:	Hours Slept:
Heart rate:	Walking time:	Blood Pressure:
How do you feel (1 being poor) circle:	**1 2 3 4 5 6 7 8 9 10**	

Notes

Daily Medication

Date ____ / ____ / ____

Medications	Morning	Afternoon	Evening
Drug & Dose:	Time:		
Drug & Dose:			
Drug & Dose:			
Drug & Dose:			
Drug & Dose:			
Drug & Dose:			
Drug & Dose:			

Daily Statistics

Weight:	Temp:	Hours Slept:
Heart rate:	Walking time:	Blood Pressure:
How do you feel (1 being poor) circle: ⟹	**1 2 3 4 5 6 7 8 9 10**	

Notes

Daily Medication

Date ____/____/____

Medications	Morning	Afternoon	Evening
Drug & Dose:	Time:		
Drug & Dose:			
Drug & Dose:			
Drug & Dose:			
Drug & Dose:			
Drug & Dose:			
Drug & Dose:			

Daily Statistics

Weight:	Temp:	Hours Slept:
Heart rate:	Walking time:	Blood Pressure:
How do you feel (1 being poor) circle:	1 2 3 4 5 6 7 8 9 10	

Notes

Daily Medication

Date ____/____/____

Medications	Morning	Afternoon	Evening
Drug & Dose:	Time:		
Drug & Dose:			
Drug & Dose:			
Drug & Dose:			
Drug & Dose:			
Drug & Dose:			
Drug & Dose:			

Daily Statistics

Weight:	Temp:	Hours Slept:
Heart rate:	Walking time:	Blood Pressure:
How do you feel (1 being poor) circle: ⟹	**1 2 3 4 5 6 7 8 9 10**	

Notes

Daily Medication

Date ____/____/____

Medications	Morning	Afternoon	Evening
Drug & Dose:	Time:		
Drug & Dose:			
Drug & Dose:			
Drug & Dose:			
Drug & Dose:			
Drug & Dose:			
Drug & Dose:			

Daily Statistics

Weight:	Temp:	Hours Slept:
Heart rate:	Walking time:	Blood Pressure:
How do you feel (1 being poor) circle: ⟹	**1 2 3 4 5 6 7 8 9 10**	

Notes

Daily Medication

Date ____/____/____

Medications		Morning	Afternoon	Evening
Drug & Dose:		Time:		
Drug & Dose:				
Drug & Dose:				
Drug & Dose:				
Drug & Dose:				
Drug & Dose:				
Drug & Dose:				

Daily Statistics

Weight:	Temp:	Hours Slept:
Heart rate:	Walking time:	Blood Pressure:
How do you feel (1 being poor) circle: ⟹	**1 2 3 4 5 6 7 8 9 10**	

Notes

Daily Medication

Date ____/____/____

Medications	Morning	Afternoon	Evening
Drug & Dose:	Time:		
Drug & Dose:			
Drug & Dose:			
Drug & Dose:			
Drug & Dose:			
Drug & Dose:			
Drug & Dose:			

Daily Statistics

Weight:	Temp:	Hours Slept:
Heart rate:	Walking time:	Blood Pressure:
How do you feel (1 being poor) circle: ⟹	**1 2 3 4 5 6 7 8 9 10**	

www.ingramcontent.com/pod-product-compliance
Lightning Source LLC
Chambersburg PA
CBHW080256180526
45167CB00006B/2548